The Living State and Cancer

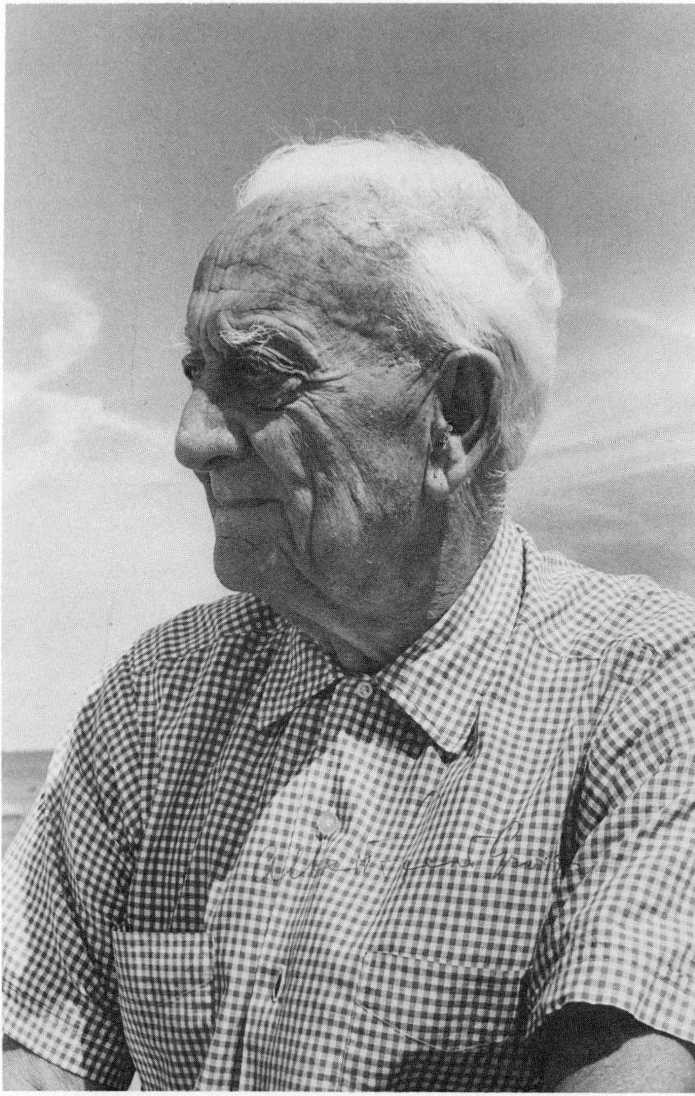

The Living State and Cancer

ALBERT SZENT-GYÖRGYI, M.D., Ph.D., N.L.

Workshop of the National Foundation for Cancer Research
Marine Biological Laboratory
Woods Hole, Massachusetts

MARCEL DEKKER, INC. New York and Basel

Library of Congress Cataloging in Publication Data

Szent-Györgyi, Albert, [Date]
The living state and cancer.

Bibliography: p.
1. Cancer. 2. Charge transfer. 3. Life (Biology)
I. Title.
RC263.S99
ISBN 0-8247-6761-6

MARCEL DEKKER, INC.
270 Madison Avenue, New York, New York 10016

Current printing (last digit):
10 9 8 7 6 5 4 3 2 1

PRINTED IN THE UNITED STATES OF AMERICA

Contents

Acknowledgments

My profound gratitude is offered to the American public for its generosity which enables me to pursue my research unencumbered by financial difficulties. My thanks are extended to Mr. Franklin C. Salisbury who volunteered to put my problem before the American public, and built the National Foundation for Cancer Research (7315 Wisconsin Avenue, Suite 851W, Bethesda, Maryland 20014). He dedicated the Foundation to the idea of stopping cancer in our lifetime.

The Living State and Cancer

1

Introduction

Ascorbic acid was discovered 50 years ago. In a remarkably short time we knew all that was worth knowing about its molecule, but its biological function remained an enigma. We must discover this function not only to satisfy our curiosity, but also because without this knowledge medicine is unable to use this remarkable substance intelligently.

That this lack of understanding has deeper roots is suggested by the fact that similar relations also exist in other fields. Cancer, for instance, and the host of degenerative diseases are still rampaging freely, causing untold suffering. Cancer research has stagnated; we do not understand cancer better than Rudolph Virchow did a century ago.

The situation is similar with "the living state." There is probably no biologist who has never asked himself, "What is life?" But, certainly, there is none who has given a satisfactory answer to this question. Science is built on the experience that Nature answers intelligent questions intelligently; thus if Nature is silent, something may be wrong with the question. The question is wrong because there is no such thing as "life"—nobody has ever seen it. What we can see are only material systems which have this wonderful quality of being alive. "Alive" is a quality, and the question is, "What quality?"

It is customary to divide the surrounding world into *animate* (alive) and *inanimate* (not alive), a division that is sharp and unequivocal. It is very rarely that we have any hesitation about the state to which something belongs. The subtle reactivity of living systems is what differentiates between the two states, the difference being so sharp that it is reasonable to suppose that it could not originate only from some unusual combination of relations, but has as its basis a different physicochemical state which can be described in terms of exact sciences. That the "living state" is a specific physical state has long been suggested by the disturbing experience of electron spin resonance (ESR) spectroscopists: All living matter, be it "your finger or the mouse's tail," gives an ESR signal, and is thus paramagnetic.

The fact that biology is unable to solve some of the most important everyday problems of medicine while harvesting the most brilliant successes in other fields, indicates that there are gaps and uncharted territories in our basic knowledge which research is unable to penetrate. Thus, our quest has to start with identifying these blank spots on the map of knowledge. To do so we have to assume the wide outlook of natural philosophy and start with reviewing the structure of living systems.

The macroscopic anatomists of the Renaissance recognized that our body is built of organs such as the liver, lung, and kidney. The microscopic anatomists of the nineteenth century showed these organs to be built of more or less independent small units called cells, the collective function of which results in our individual life. In the latter half of the nineteenth century it was recognized that these cells consist of molecules into which the cells can be decomposed. This made biology into a "molecular biology," which has harvested the most brilliant successes.

Molecules, in turn, can be decomposed into atoms, and atoms into electrons and atomic nuclei. The physics of the twentieth century has shown that atomic nuclei and electrons are complex systems of still smaller units into which they can be decomposed.

We do not know how far this subdivisibility of Nature continues. The biologist has reached his limits with atomic nuclei and electrons. Further decomposition into still smaller units demands enormous energies which are far beyond biological dimensions.

To sum up, there are four dimensions with which the biologist must be concerned: macroscopic, microscopic, molecular, and submolecular or electronic. Biology readily followed physics into the first three, but took practically no cognizance of the fourth; it stopped at the molecular level, though its way into the submolecular or electronic level was paved by pioneers such as the Pullmans, P.-O. Löwdin and others.

Our senses were developed by Nature to enable us to get through the day alive, find what we need, and distinguish between a dog and a bear before being eaten. By "understanding" we mean having experienced something similar. Thus, since our senses were formed for the macroscopic dimension we could have no experience of the submolecular. Molecules are on the borderline of the two dimensions. A sodium chloride molecule is more or less the same substance as the salt we have on our dinner table. The situation is different with the submolecular or electronic dimension. This is an entirely alien world about which we have no personal experience whatsoever, which we cannot "understand." That science could penetrate into it at all is due to the fact that its tool, mathematics, is valid for all dimensions. The rules and regulations of this world are dealt with by quantum or wave mechanics and are often contrary to our everyday experience.

It was at an early date that I began to feel that the wonderful subtlety of biological reactions could not be produced solely by molecules, but had to be produced partly by much smaller and more mobile units which could hardly be anything else than electrons. The main actors of life had to be electrons whereas the clumsy and unreactive protein molecules had to be the stage on which the drama of life was enacted. Electrons, to be mobile, need a conductor, which led me to the conclusion that proteins have to be electronic conductors. Toward the end of the 1930s theories began to appear about the submolecular structure of condensed matter. This opened the possibility of electronic mobility in proteins, and thus in 1941 I proposed that proteins may be conductors.

My proposition was unanimously rejected. The more lenient critics called it a "lame duck," and the more severe ones called it a "dead duck." Two apparently convincing objections were raised. Firstly, by that time a great number of proteins had been isolated and thoroughly studied, and none of them had shown any signs of conductivity. Secondly, semiconduction had been found a satisfactory explanation and proteins did not fit into it. It was shown that semiconduction was brought about by the proximity of the "valence" and "conduction band" which made it possible for heat agitation to excite electrons from the former to the latter. In proteins the two bands were found to be too far from one another for such excitation.

Many years passed before it occurred to me that my critics had actually put the clue into my hand and shown the way to the verification of my theory. Proteins had to be in the living state only in vivo, in the living cell. If my theory were correct, proteins could no longer be in the living state after having been extracted, isolated, purified, and crystallized, but had to behave as inanimate objects do. Further, if semiconduction was produced by exciting electrons from the valence band to the conduction band, then Nature could have produced conduction in proteins by simply transferring electrons from their valence band to other molecules by "charge transfer" (see later).

2

Proteins

The basic blueprints of life are guarded by the nucleic acids, while the business of life is carried on by the proteins. The proteins are long chains of peptide bonds held together by single carbon atoms, the α-carbon atoms of the constituent amino acids. The peptide bonds are flat, planar structures consisting of three atoms, a carbon, nitrogen, and oxygen, held together by bonds which are neither single nor double but something in between.

Crystallographic measurements show the double link between C and O (Fig. 1) to be longer and the single bond between C and N shorter, as such bonds usually are, which means that the two bonds are neither double nor single, but something between the two. These bonds could be looked upon as a mixture of the two resonating mesomeric forms, (a) and (b). According to L. Pauling (1970) the mixture consists of 60% (a) and 40% (b), and there is a difference of 21 kcal in the energy of the two. The bonds could be symbolized by Figure 1c which indicates that there is no free rotation around the C–N bond to disturb the planar structure.*

The peptide bonds have π electrons. If we use "P" as the notation for the peptide bond, then the structure of the protein can be symbolized as ...PCPCPCPCPC..., where

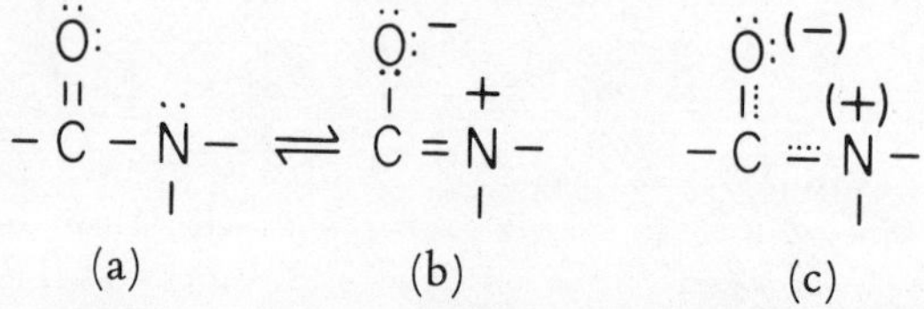

Figure 1 Mesomeric forms of peptide bonds.

the "side groups" hang out sideways, linked to the C atoms. This threadlike molecule can take up the most varied shapes by folding. The final result of this linkage is macromolecules, which are often built of subunits, and have a molecular weight of thousands or millions of daltons.

In a pure protein all orbitals are occupied by electron pairs held firmly in their place by their nucleus, the two electrons of the pairs spinning in opposite directions, strongly coupled, and compensating each other's magnetic moments. The final result is a dielectric "closed shell" molecule of low reactivity which has no electronic mobility.

Every atom has its own energy levels, the lower ones of which are occupied by electrons. Over the occupied levels are empty unoccupied levels. In condensed matter (i.e., solids), the energy levels of similar atoms come to lie close to one another. Since the exclusion principle allows only two electrons to have the same energy (and this only if the two electrons have an opposite spin) the electrons perturb one another and the energy levels split up. The final result is a bundle of energy levels, an "energy band" in which there are no empty energy levels which would offer room for motion. W. Shockley (1950) compared the situation in such a band with a completely filled parking lot in which no motion is possible.

The outer "valence electrons" form the *valence band* which is the highest occupied band. The empty energy levels which lie over the occupied ones also form bands, the lowest of which, next to the valence band, is called the *conduction band.* This band is so termed because in semiconductors the valence band and the conduction band lie so close to one another that the energy of heat agitation suffices to raise ("excite") electrons from the former to the latter, on which the electron finds room for motion ("conduction"). Semiconduction is thus *conduction in the excited state.*

In proteins the valence band and the conduction band are too far from one another to make it possible for heat agitation to raise electrons from the former to the latter. Pure proteins are thus not semiconductors. They consist of clumsy macromolecules of low reactivity with no electronic mobility. Such a molecule could not perform the wonderfully subtle reactions of living systems. Thus our problem boils down to the question: Is there a way in which such a molecule could acquire a higher degree of reactivity and an electronic mobility?

There is a way. It consists of taking electrons out of the valence band and thereby create empty places and room for motion. In the same way as the removal of a single car from a filled parking lot makes all the rest mobile, so in the valence band the removal of electrons makes all the other electrons mobile too. As mentioned earlier, in semiconductors mobility and conductivity are created by exciting electrons into the conduction band. In proteins conductivity can thus be created by taking out electrons from the valence band also without excitation. This can be done by *charge transfer,* the transfer of electrons from the protein to another molecule whereby the protein acts as *electron donor*, and the other molecule as *electron acceptor.* The resulting conduction is then a *conduction in the ground state.* The acceptor may be present as an "acceptor impurity," as proposed by L. Brillouin (1962).

Energy bands may seem an abstraction, but many phenomena of our everyday life are due to them; for example, radio, television, and computers are based on them. Metals such as copper are good electric conductors because their valence bands are but partially filled, and there is plenty of room for motion. Insulators may also have their energy bands, provided the bands are completely filled and the conduction band is too far from the valence band to allow excitation to it, the *forbidden zone* between the two being too wide.

Whereas conductivity can be created by taking electrons out of the valence band, by *desaturating* it electronically, reactivity can be induced by taking out electrons one by one. When taking out single electrons, electron pairs have to be separated, uncoupled. The electron remaining behind is left uncoupled, on a half-occupied orbital, which upsets the balance of the whole molecule. The place of the eliminated electron is then taken by an *electron hole.* Molecules containing one or more uncoupled electrons are called *free radicals*, and these are known to be very reactive. If more than one electron is eliminated, a multiradical is generated. As is shown later, our body is built to a great extent of such radicals. Uncoupled electrons and free radicals can be easily detected by the signal they give in the ESR spectroscope. The conduction generated by taking out electrons is a "p" type conduction, the charge carriers being positive holes.

Needless to say, there is no such thing as "the

protein," for proteins are exceedingly versatile substances which fulfill the very different functions within our body. Some of these functions may be passive and very simple, primitive, and demand no conductivity or reactivity. The main function of serum albumin, for instance, is to maintain the osmotic pressure of blood. Collagen fibers fulfill their function simply with their tensile strength. None of these functions demands conductivity or a high reactivity. On the other hand, many of our complex functions are brought about by the collective action of protein molecules which would be impossible without a high reactivity and conductivity.

Electronic mobility opens the possibility of transmission of messages, information, and energy, as well as an integration of function. When a protein molecule is desaturated electronically by charge transfer the real donor is not a nitrogen atom of an NH_2 group, but the valence band. So the electron deficiency may be distributed over the whole band.

At the side of conductivity and reactivity, protein molecules have another quality which is most important for life and the building of its structures: cohesiveness. Cohesive forces are often summed up under the name of "van der Waals interactions." These forces are derived from two different sources, one of which is dipolar attractions, the other the London quantum mechanical dispersion forces. The former are long-range forces that decrease with the square of the distance, whereas the latter are short-distance forces that decrease with a much higher power of the distance. These forces are important for holding the cells and cellular structure together.

K. Laki and J. Ladik (1976), at one of the workshops of the NFCR, made the important discovery that the cohesive forces depend greatly on the electronic desaturation of the protein. With increasing desaturation they may increase by several orders of magnitude. As is shown later, in cancer desaturation is of a low degree and as a consequence cohesive forces have to be low, which may be responsible for the lack of "contact inhibition" and for the ease with which cancer spreads, leading to its most feared complication, metastasis. D. R. Coman (1944), in his classical experiments, actually measured the cohesive forces holding cells together. He found the cohesive forces to be very low in cancer.

---

*Fascinating possibilities are opened up for biology by the fact that the (b) form of the peptide bond has a dipole character, even if the axis of the dipole does not coincide with the axis of the peptide chain. We could symbolize the peptide chain as shown in Figure 1a or 1b. The single units can be described as superpositions of the two mesomeric structures. A dipole structure induced by an external effect on one site could induce a dipole character in the peptide bond on the other sites. The dipole character induced in the last peptide bond of the chain could induce a dipole character in the whole chain. Thus messages and information could be propagated through the whole peptide. Also, sonic modes of vibration, stretching or shortening the double bond, may lead to transition from one resonant form to the other.

If we denote the structure in Figure 2b by 0 and denote the dipole structure in Figure 2a by 1, then,

Figure 2 Polar and nonpolar forms of peptide chains.

together these constitute a system of two digits, 0 and 1, which may play an important role in memory and learning.

These possibilities may currently be no more than products of imagination, but may shed unexpected new light on the mechanism of memory and learning, and the mysteries of protein, introducing new periodicities on the electronic level.

3

Acceptor-Donor Relations

Methylglyoxal and Glyoxalase

Mendeleev, in his periodic chart of the atoms, has brought the known elements into one coherent system. What underlies this system is the fact that the electrons surrounding the atomic nucleus form shells and these shells tend to assume the structure of a noble gas. The elements on the left side of the chart have more, the elements on the right side have fewer electrons than the nearest noble gas. Consequently, the elements on the left tend to give off electrons, that is, act as electron donors, while the elements on the right tend to take up electrons, that is, act as acceptors. The elements in the middle do neither. What drives the electrons over from the donor to the acceptor side is the trend of Nature to decrease free energy and increase entropy. So when electrons are passed from donor to acceptor energy will be liberated and entropy will be increased. It is this that drives life.

The strongest acceptor is the element in the top row on the extreme right of the chart, fluorine. There may be many reasons why Nature did not base the energetics of life on fluorine. One of these, which suffices as an explanation, is that there is very little fluorine. The acceptor underlying the energetics of life has to be ubiquitous. Similar considerations may hold for the other halogens, and so the next best choice was the element in the top row of the next column, which is oxygen. Oxygen is the universal electron acceptor of the biosphere.

The strongest electron donor is the element in the top row on the extreme left of the chart, which is hydrogen. When H and O interact, water (H_2O) is formed, and a great quantity of energy is liberated. This energy is the fuel of life. A mixture of H and O reaches its energy minimum in the formation of water, and once water is formed, no more energy can be liberated. To produce an acceptor the H and O had to be separated.

The living state is the electronically desaturated state of protein. When life originated, three and a half billion years ago, our globe was covered by a dense layer of water vapor. There was no light and no oxygen near its surface. Electron acceptors could thus be produced only by separating H and O inside molecules, by shifting the H atoms to one end, and the O atoms to the other end of the molecules. A carbohydrate is a molecule containing carbon and elements of water, corresponding to the general formula $C_nH_{2n}O_n$. The simplest carbohydrate is formaldehyde, CH_2O. There is no way to separate the H atoms from the O atom inside this simple molecule. The next higher carbohydrate is glycolaldehyde, $C_2H_4O_2$, which leads to acetaldehyde, which has the H atoms at one end and the O atom on the other. This single aldehydic O, which in the presence of water is strongly hydrated, is a very weak acceptor, too weak to desaturate protein. The next higher carbohydrate is glyceraldehyde, $C_3H_6O_3$ (Fig. 3a). If a water molecule is taken out of it and the place of the eliminated water is taken by two H atoms, methylglyoxal (MG) results (Fig. 3b). MG has the O atoms on one end, and H atoms on the other end of its molecule, and is a strong acceptor. It has in its ketonic O a low-lying orbital (Abdulnur, 1976) on which it can accommodate an additional electron. It has a highly reactive aldehydic group with which it can attack protein. Nature is simple but subtle. The π systems of its two conjugated double bonds fuse to a big π system. MG is the universal electron

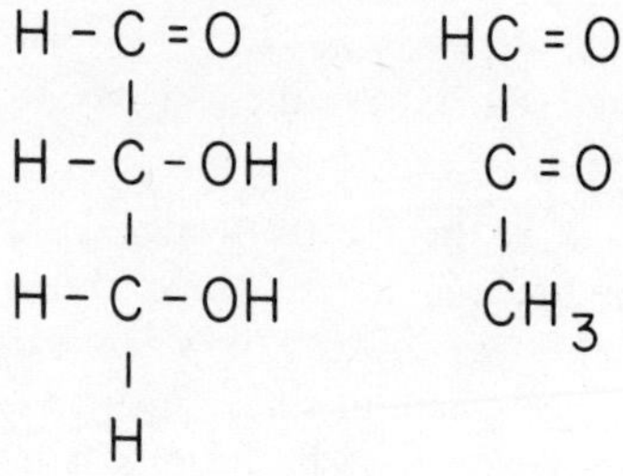

(a) (b)

Figure 3 (a) Glyceraldehyde; (b) methylglyoxal.

acceptor of the biosphere for reversible reactions. Taking out electrons irreversibly means killing. For this end Nature uses aromatic carbonyls, which are used in the vegetable world in defense against invading bacteria.

That MG plays some important role in Nature was indicated by the fact that more than 60 years ago two British and a German biochemist (Dakin and Dudley, 1913; Neuberg, 1913) discovered an apparently ubiquitous and most active enzyme, glyoxalase, which could transform methylglyoxal at an amazing rate into D-lactic acid. F. G. Hopkins and E. J. Morgan (1948) have shown glyoxalase to be an enzymatic system rather than a single enzyme, which consists of two enzymes called glyoxalase I and glyoxalase II. K. Lohmann (1932) showed this enzymatic system to use SH-glutathione as coenzyme. MG and SH-glutathione spontaneously form a hemimercaptal which is the substrate of glyoxalase I. Glyoxalase I shifts the two H atoms from the aldehydic end to the ketonic O,

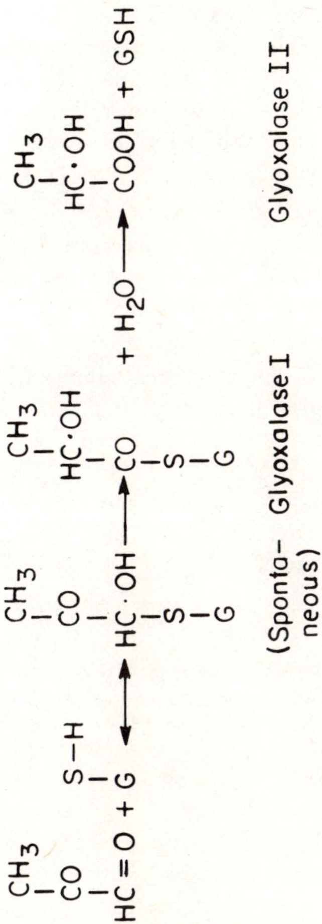

Figure 4 Action mechanism of glyoxalase.

thereby transforming the hemimercaptal into a thioester. The glyoxalase II then splits the ester into D-lactic acid and free glutathione, recovering the coenzyme (Yamazoye, 1936; Racker, 1951, 1952). The entire process is summed up in Figure 4. The transfer number of glyoxalase I is 40,000, whereas that of glyoxalase II is only 10,000. Nature seems to be in a hurry only to inactivate the MG, and does the final splitting more leisurely; thus the tissues may contain some thioester.

In spite of this detailed knowledge, the real function of glyoxalase is still a mystery, since neither MG nor D-lactic acid is known to lie on a metabolic highway. Acting as electron acceptor in the desaturation of protein would fully account for its existence.

Methylglyoxal can be formed along various metabolic pathways. It can even form spontaneously from glyceraldehyde by the loss of one molecule of water. As shown by V. Riddle and F. W. Lorenz (1968), this reaction is catalyzed by polyvalent anions, such as phosphate, and is catalyzed, as discovered by A. Bonsignore and his associates (1977), by lysine.

MG can be called an *acceptor impurity of protein*. It was L. Brillouin who proposed first that the valence band of protein may be desaturated electronically by "acceptor impurities," thereby bringing new energy levels into the system.

4

The α and β State

Transformation

As with all other chemical reactions, charge transfer is driven by the trend of Nature to decrease free energy and increase entropy. Molecules contain an equal number of positive and negative charges, are thus electroneutral. In charge transfer, which consists of electrons being transferred from one molecule to another, this parity is broken. Charge transfer has to work against an electric gradient. As a consequence, the transferred electron will remain attracted by the donor molecule and will oscillate between donor and acceptor, spending various lengths of time on each one depending on the difference of the energy level of donor and acceptor orbitals. If the electron spends only a part of its time on the acceptor, as is usually the case, it is customary to say that only part of the electron, say one-tenth or one-hundredth of it, was transferred. Charge transfer can thus have very different levels and, accordingly, the electronic desaturation and living state of the protein can also have very different levels. With a low degree of desaturation only a very primitive form of life could have developed.

At the rate at which our globe cooled, its water vapor envelope condensed. Eventually, light could reach its surface. What life did with this light was to capture its photons and use their free energy and negative entropy for the separation of the elements of water, producing hydrogen and oxygen. Oxygen is a very strong acceptor, ready to accept a whole electron. Its appearance thus opened the possibility of a high degree of desaturation in protein and a correspondingly high degree of development and differentiation, leading to increasingly complex and subtle biological reactions.

The appearance of light and oxygen cuts the history of life into two periods, the first of which I have called the α, and the second the β period. In the anaerobic and dark α period there was no free oxygen. Life had to depend for the desaturation of protein on the acceptors it could produce out of its own material, first on MG, to which it could transfer only relatively small parts of electrons. Correspondingly, in the α period only simple, primitive living forms of life could be developed, forms which have left behind but very few traces. The main function of these organisms had to be an unbridled proliferation which made life perennial. Proliferation had to be favored by the simplicity of structures and the weakness of cohesion.

In the β period oxygen made the transfer of larger parts of electrons, or even whole electrons, possible. With the higher degree of desaturation thus achieved, life started to develop and differentiate, and produce increasingly complex structures capable of increasingly complex and subtle functions. The development of structures and the increased cohesion which held these structures together must have interfered with proliferation. Whereas the anaerobic and dark α period was the period of unbridled proliferation, the β period was the period of development and differentiation, in which cell division was subjected to regulation.

The importance of these relations is in the fact that there has to be cell division in the β period also, but to be able to divide the cell has to reduce cohesiveness and dismount part of its structures, that is, dedifferentiate. In order to be able to divide, the cell must return, to some extent, to the α state. This is why all dividing cells resemble one another, and cancer cells are closely akin to embryonic cells, or any other dividing cell, the similarity going as far as the production of fetal proteins.

The α state is the ground state of life. The most stable state of any system is at the minimum of free energy and the maximum of entropy, and this is the α state. If the cellular organization becomes unstable, the cell will return to the proliferative α state, and stay there. The more complete this return to the α state, the more unbridled will the ensuing proliferation be, the looser the structure, and the greater the tendency of the resulting tumor to spread, that is, the greater will be its malignancy. In a way, the cancer cell is not a sick cell. Its vitality, as that of a wild type, may even be higher than that of a normal cell.

5

Permittivity

In 1949 I found that vital functions, such as contractility, could be preserved by keeping the material at a low temperature in 50% glycerol. The psoas muscle of the rabbit could, even after years of storage, develop the maximum tension it had ever displayed in vivo. The method was later used by others to conserve the motility of sperm, and now plays a major role in animal husbandry, via artificial insemination. Subsequently, glycerol was used also for the preservation of blood in blood banks, until C. E. Huggins (1963) replaced glycerol with dimethyl sulfoxide. These activities were a mystery, for neither glycerol nor dimethyl sulfoxide is "physiological." The conserving action was ascribed first to the low temperature, and the glycerol and dimethyl sulfoxide were thought to act simply by preventing freezing. It was clear to me, however, that these fluids had some other quality to which they owed their conserving action. Charge transfer led me to the dielectric constant, ϵ.

The dielectric constant of a substance is defined as the relation of the capacitance of two condenser plates, with the space between them filled by a vacuum or the material in question. The quality of a substance, induced by its ϵ, is "permittivity." A high ϵ means a high permittivity, a low ϵ low permittivity.

The permittivity of a fluid depends in the first place on the charge, dipole moment, and mobility of its particles. A solvent of high ϵ will more easily depolarize the electric field surrounding an electrically charged point than one of a low ϵ. It is evident that a process (such as charge transfer) which involves changes in charge distribution will have to depend greatly on the ϵ of the medium.

Charge transfer involves the separation of positive and negative charges, that is, the separation of an electron from the positive hole it leaves behind. This separation will be facilitated by a medium of high dielectric constant, such as water, and will be disfavored by substances of low ϵ, such as alcohol. The opposite is true for polymerization which is due to the mutual attraction of oppositely charged points of the polymerizing particles. If, in Figure 5, the top line represents a charge transfer complex in which the positive and negative charges were separated and displaced to the ends, then it is evident that a dimerization, as shown in the bottom part of the figure, will facilitate charge transfer, and, vice versa, that charge transfer will facilitate polymerization. A medium of high ϵ will depolarize the charges and so will inhibit polymerization, or make the polymer dissociate. In some fluids there will be no charge transfer at all, the permittivity being too low to allow separation of charges, or too high to allow polymerization.

Methylgloxal and methylamine, when mixed, form a charge transfer complex which is yellow in an aqueous and red in an alcohol solution (ethanol ϵ = 26; methanol ϵ = 33). The explanation is that in water (ϵ = 81,5) the single particles of the complex show an absorption in the near ultraviolet, whereas in alcohol they associate to a polymer

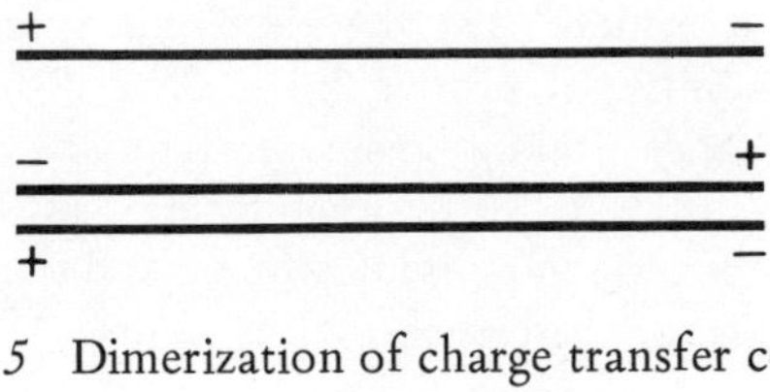

Figure 5 Dimerization of charge transfer complex.

which has an absorption around 475 nm. The measurements of the molecular weight by H. Pohl (unpublished observations) indicated that a tetramer was formed. The absorption of the yellow monomer gave a very narrow peak, indicating a strong electronic delocalization, while the absorption of the red alcohol solution was wider, indicating strong localization of the mutually attracting charges. The difference in color was what started me off on my study of charge transfer.

The ϵ of a medium can be altered not only by changing the chemistry of the medium but also by altering its physical state, by immobilizing its particles, which decreases the ϵ. The ϵ of water, for instance, is 81.5, whereas that of ice is 3, close to that of paraffin wax (2.1).

This is of primary import for life, the medium of which is water. Water consists of dipoles and near solid surfaces water assumes an "icelike" character, its dipoles becoming oriented. F. W. Cope (1974), R. Damadian (1971), and C. Hazlewood (1969), by measuring the relaxation time of water in tissues by nuclear magnetic resonance, found that the water of tissues was structured to a great extent. The early experiments indicated 50% structured water in cells, but the later experiments of C. Hazlewood indicated an even higher degree of structuralization. Structure means immobilization, a decrease of ϵ. This makes it evident that the electronic changes in the immediate vicinity of protein have to be different from analogous changes taking place in random water. The division of ions into "structure forming" and "structure destroying" ions is common knowledge, and thus ions may also have a major influence on the course of electronic reactions. The changes in permittivity, induced by structuralization, can be of prime import for biological processes; they allow change in the ϵ without exchanging the medium.

The experiment reproduced in Table 1 clearly brings out the importance of ϵ for charge transfer and the resulting electronic distribution. In this experiment a series of test tubes were filled with various solvents diluted with different amounts of water. The first tube contained no water at all, the second 10%, the third 20%, and soon, until the last tube contained only pure water. Then a drop of 40% methylglyoxal and a drop of 40% methylamine were added and the intensity of the developing red color was noted by crosses after 10 min of storage. Red color meant the formation of the polymerized charge transfer complex. The various organic solvents used had a considerably lower ϵ than water and so the ϵ of their mixture increased from 0 to 100%. Table 1 points out the antagonism between a high and low ϵ. As the table shows, the strongest polymerization and charge transfer were obtained in glycerol, which explains its mysterious preserving action. The high viscosity and hydrophylic nature of glycerol may have contributed to the effect, by decreasing its mobility.

The second best medium was methanol, followed by ethanol, but these solvents cannot be used for conserving tissues because they denature protein. The ϵ of anhydrous acetone is evidently too low, but acetone can be made into a good medium by adding water, which thereby increases its ϵ of 25. The permittivity of pure dimethyl sulfoxide and dimethylformamide is too low to allow the separation

Table 1 Production of Colored Charge Transfer Complexes of MG and Methylamine in Various Solvents[a]

% WATER —	0	10	20	30	40	50	60	70	80	90	100
METHANOL	+++	+++	+++	+++	(+++)	++	(++)	(++)	+	(+)	±
ETHANOL	+++	(++)	(++)	++	++	(++)	(++)	+	(+)	(+)	±
PROPYLALCOHOL	++	++	++	++	+	+	(+)	±	0	0	±
ACETONE	0	++	++	+	∓	±	0	0	0	0	±
ETHYLENEGLYCOL	0	0	0	0	0	0	±	+	(++)	(++)	±
GLYCEROL	+++	++++	++++	++++	++++	+++	+++	++	++	+	±
DIMETHYLSULFOXIDE	0	±	(+)	+	++	+++	++	+	+	±	±
DIMETHYLFORMAMIDE	0	(±)	±	+	(++)	++	++	++	+	(+)	±
FORMAMIDE	0	0	0	0	0	0	0	0	0	(±)	±
DIOXANE	0	0	0	0	0	0	0	0	0	0	±

[a]Intensity of color noted by + signs. Parentheses mean less color. For details see text.

of charges while that of water is too high to allow polymerization. Between the two extremes is a transitory zone in which both processes are possible. In dimethyl sulfoxide the maximum was reached at 50%, in dimethylformamide it was reached at 60%. (The ϵ of dimethyl sulfoxide is 45, that of dimethylformamide is somewhat lower, 37.) Formamide has a very high ϵ (109) and, accordingly, no charge transfer was observed in it. The same is true for dioxane. The optimal permittivity seems to be at around $\epsilon = 65$. Narcosis by agents such as ether or chloroform may be due to their lowering ϵ.

As experience with muscle contraction shows, permittivity is a most important quality from a biological point of view. In some respects it parallels pH, although until now it has been disregarded. I cannot remember having seen permittivity discussed in any textbook of biological chemistry, and it is rarely mentioned in discussions on constants, a natural consequence of the neglect afforded the whole electronic dimension.

6

Methylglyoxal and NH_2

Methylglyoxal interacts with proteins by means of its aldehydic C=O, with which it attacks primary amino NH_2 groups. Since proteins are very complex, I started the study of this interaction by collecting experience on models in which aliphatic amines took the place of protein. The simplest aliphatic amine is methylamine, CH_3NH_2. Proteins have NH_2 in their lysine and arginine residues. The NH_2 groups of lysine are at the end of a four-carbon chain (Fig. 6), which hangs out of the polypeptide as a side group. The aliphatic amine which is most similar to this side chain formation is butylamine, $C_4H_9NH_2$.

If a solution of MG and an amine is mixed, the fluid turns yellow or red, depending on the permittivity of the solvent. The yellow product obtained in water is a Schiff base, and the red color obtained in solvents of low permit-

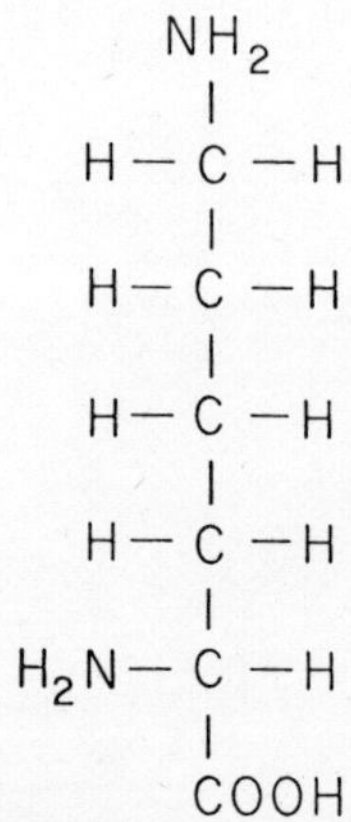

Figure 6 Lysine.

tivity is due to the polymerization of the Schiff bases. This polymerization is inhibited by water. (Only if the reagents are applied in a high concentration is a red polymer obtained in water.)

The Schiff base is not the primary product of the reaction, as can be shown by mixing a 0.2 M aqueous solution of MG and butylamine. The primary product precipitates in the form of a colorless substance which, on storage, becomes reddish-yellow. In this case polymerization is inhibited by the water, but the precipitate itself offers an anhydrous medium. The primary colorless product is, in all probability, a hemiacetal which then turns into a Schiff base by giving off a molecule of water:

$$RNH_2 + O = CHR \rightleftarrows R\underset{H}{N}-\underset{H}{\overset{OH}{C}}-R \rightarrow RN = \overset{H}{C}-R + H_2O$$

The same colorless intermediary can also be observed if a 0.5 M acetone solution of MG and CH_3NH_2 is mixed. The colorless precipitate formed turns purple within seconds. The resinous purple precipitate can be separated on the table centrifuge and changes into a purple glass on drying.

The yellow color of the Schiff base is due to the chromogenic C=N link which holds the MG and amine together, which has a strong light absorption in the near ultraviolet, spilling over into the visible. The purple color of the polymer formed in solvents of low permittivity is due to an

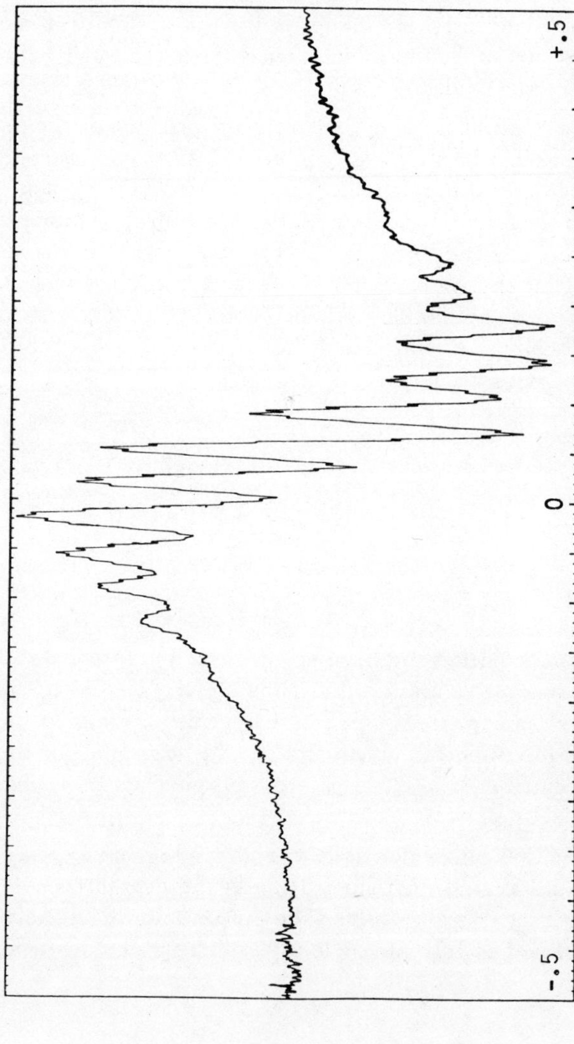

Figure 7 ESR spectrum of charge transfer complex of methylamine and methylglyoxal.

absorption which has its maximum at around 475 nm. The red color and absorption at 475 nm indicate polymerization.

In the ESR spectroscope the purple substance formed by methylamine and MG gave a strong signal with a hyperfine structure indicating charge transfer (Fig. 7). It readily dissolved in methanol or water without losing color. Though not formed in water, once formed in acetone, it retains its purple color in water for some time, even in the presence of HCl. The purple color indicates that the charge transfer complex has not dissociated. The ESR signal given by the purple substance was a surprise, because, as a rule charge transfer complexes give signals only after they have dissociated into the ionic form, into two separate radicals in which coupling is broken.

Secondary butylamine forms only a yellow Schiff base, no red polymer, for the loose ends of its molecule interfere with polymerization. The same is true for lysine.

According to K. Takahashi (1977), arginine readily interacts with MG. No colored Schiff bases are formed in this interaction, the nature of which is not understood and demands further study.

The reactions of protein and MG are but partially explained by these reactions. If powdered casein is suspended in a neutral 0.1 M watery solution of 0.1 M MG, and the suspension is incubated overnight, the casein turns yellow, which is evidently due to the formation of Schiff bases by the NH_2 groups of the lysine residues. If the NH_2 groups of casein are exhaustively acetylated, the casein remains perfectly colorless on treatment with MG. If the casein is suspended in a 0.1 M methanol solution of MG, it turns

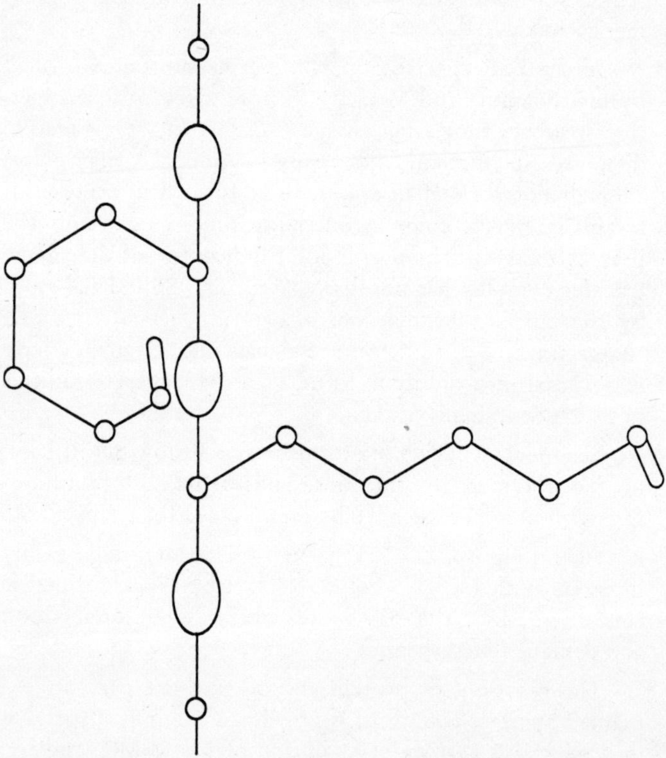

Figure 8 Peptide chain with lysine side chains, straight and folded, with attached methylglyoxal. Small rings stand for C atoms, big ovals for peptide links.

brown, that is, it assumes the color of liver. This dark color indicates complexing. Since the Schiff bases formed at the ends of the side chains could not complex with one another, they had to complex with a neighboring peptide bond of the protein. J. Ladik (1978) showed that the folding of the side chain brings the Schiff base in touch with a neighboring peptide bond, opening the possibility of charge transfer between the two (Fig. 8), which can lead to the desaturation of the valence band of the protein. As shown by J. Ladik (unpublished observations), Schiff bases are still good acceptors, almost as good as free MG. Both the Schiff bases and the peptide bonds are planar and so can establish the close contact required by charge transfer. The structuralization of the water around the protein has to decrease its permittivity, promoting this association between Schiff base and peptide bond.

As shown by R. Pethig and myself (1977), the brown casein has an increased electronic conductivity, indicating a desaturation of its valence band. This conductivity was demonstrated in even more detail by S. Bone et al. (1978).

The brown casein, washed with methanol and dried, gave a strong ESR signal at g 2 (Fig. 9). The number of spins was about one per casein molecule. J. McLaughlin and P. Gascoyne in their present, yet unpublished work, measured the quantity of the MG bound by the casein by weighing the dried samples. The results indicated that one to two MG molecules bound per lysine residue, depending on the concentration of MG. One of these may have been bound by arginine residues.

The color of the MG-treated casein or serum albumin is very similar to that of a bloodless liver, suggesting that

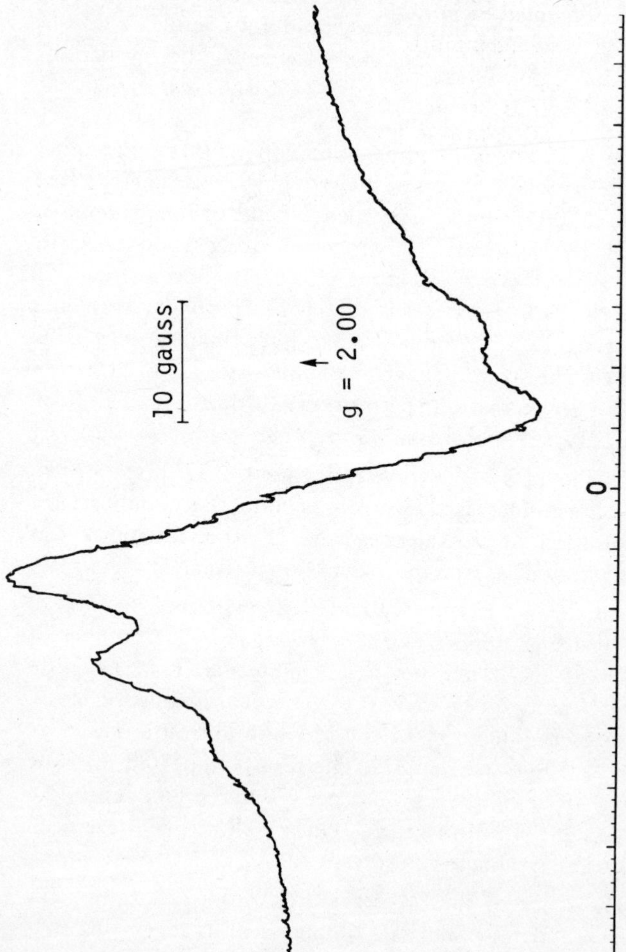

Figure 9 ESR spectrum of casein treated with methylglyoxal.

hitherto unidentified color of the liver is actually due to a complex formed by protein with MG. The brown color of the liver is such a familiar sight that no questions are asked about its origin. When, as a student, I asked my professors why the liver is brown the usual answer I obtained was, "Because it is the liver."

The carbonyl bound to the liver protein was identified by G. Fodor et al. (1978) as methylglyoxal. In these experiments the liver protein was "washed" by reprecipitating it from water at pH 4.5, and then treating the liver with strong HCl in the presence of dinitrophenylhydrazine. The hydrazones formed were isolated and identified as hydrazones of MG.

The various proteins tested, casein, lysozyme, fibrinogen, and serum albumin, containing lysine residues, all behaved similarly to casein and gave a brown derivative with MG.

Electron spectroscopists were often puzzled by the fact that all living tissues give ESR signals. These signals were ascribed to unidentified free radicals formed in metabolism. The foregoing experiments suggested that the signals might be due to radicals formed by proteins. In order to decide whether the signals given by liver tissue were radicals formed by the soluble or insoluble structure-forming proteins, mouse livers were blended in ice-cold half-saturated ammonium sulfate (Pohl et al., 1977) solutions. Soluble radicals were expected to stay in solution while the structural proteins precipitated and were separated on the centrifuge. The proteins of the supernate were precipitated by 100% saturation with $(NH_4)_2SO_4$. These latter gave only a very weak signal, whereas the

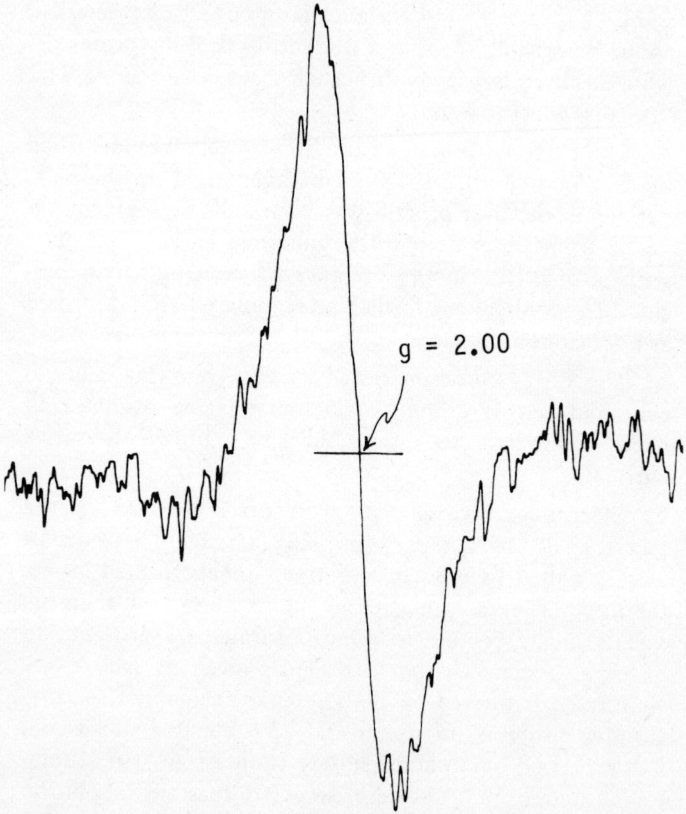

Figure 10 ESR signal of structure proteins of liver, soluble in 50% $(NH_4)_2SO_4$.

precipitate containing the structural proteins of the tissue gave a strong signal (Fig. 10). This confirms the conclusion that the greatest part of the ESR signal of live tissues is due to the radical nature of the proteins of the cellular structures.

Analogous preparations made from a parenchymal rat liver carcinoma gave but very poor signal which could not always be clearly distinguished from noise. Whereas structures of normal liver are built of radicals, those of the tumor seem to be built more of closed shell molecules.

In charge transfer two electrically charged free radicals are formed, the donor with a positive, the acceptor with a negative charge. Charged free radicals are extremely reactive and it is doubtful whether their existence is compatible with life. When making the protein conductant by charge transfer, Nature avoids this difficulty by incorporating the acceptor, MG, into the protein first, and transferring charges onto it after. This way the charges produced remain in the same molecule which, though transformed into a biradical, has no net charge. The whole process is very similar to the *doping* by which germanium and silicon are made into strong conductors in semiconductor industry. Nature discovered doping billions of years before man did.

Why, of all organs, only the liver and kidney are brown is a matter of conjecture. Both organs are seats of strong energy changes and are exposed to powerful streams, the liver to those of our digested food, the kidney to those of the urine. It is understandable if Nature tied the MG strongly to the protein. The relative lack of color in other organs does not mean that they have no MG. As is shown later, MG also produces a relatively colorless charge transfer complex with NH_2 groups, a complex that absorbs in the near ultraviolet. We do our thinking with the "gray matter" of our brain and gray is diluted black. So the brain is not lacking color. Of course, all tissues contain many different colored substances, such as carotenes, flavines, cytochromes, to name a few, but the colors discussed cannot be entirely due to them.

All structural proteins contain lysine. The protein carries with it the chemical mechanism of its own electronic desaturation.

7

Ascorbic Acid

Ascorbic acid was discovered half a century ago, and in a remarkably short time we knew everything about its structure that was worth knowing. Contrary to this, its biological function remained a mystery. Since we can control only what we understand, medicine was unable to make full use of ascorbic acid. There is confusion even about simple questions, such as the daily dose of ascorbic acid needed to maintain health. While some of its students, such as I. Stone (1972) and L. Pauling (1970), advocate megadoses, the small U.S. Recommended Dietary Allowance of 60 mg has been reduced to 45 mg/day.

If a dilute, 0.1 M aqueous solution of MG and methylamine is mixed, a slowly developing yellow color indicates the formation of a Schiff base. In the presence of ascorbic acid a red color appears and rapidly deepens, absorbing at 475 nm. In the ESR spectroscope the mixture of methylamine and MG gives a strong and complex signal (Fig. 11). Ascorbic acid makes the signal much stronger without changing its character. All this indicates that ascorbic acid is involved in this charge transfer.

A neutral ascorbic acid solution in contact with air gives a typical ESR signal, a doublet with a coupling constant of 1.7 G, each part of the doublet consisting of a triplet with a coupling constant of 0.17 (Fig. 12), as described by earlier workers (e.g., Yamazaki et al., 1960; Lagerkrantz, 1964; Kirano and Kwan, 1972). The signal appears very rapidly on admission of air to an anaerobic solution.

As shown by P. Gascoyne (unpublished observations), if MG is added to the solution of the radical of ascorbate, the ESR signal disappears, indicating a reaction between

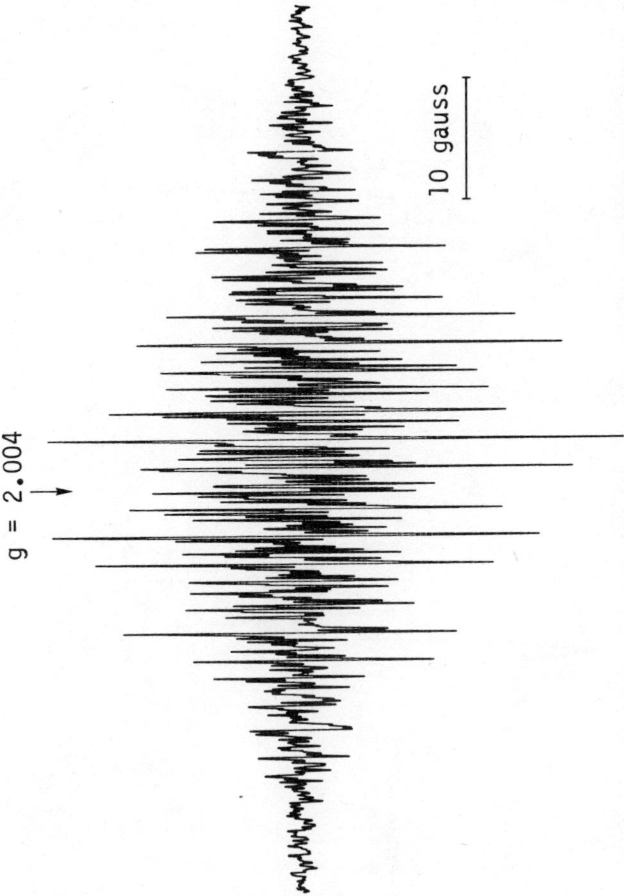

Figure 11 ESR spectrum of a mixture of methylamine and methylglyoxal.

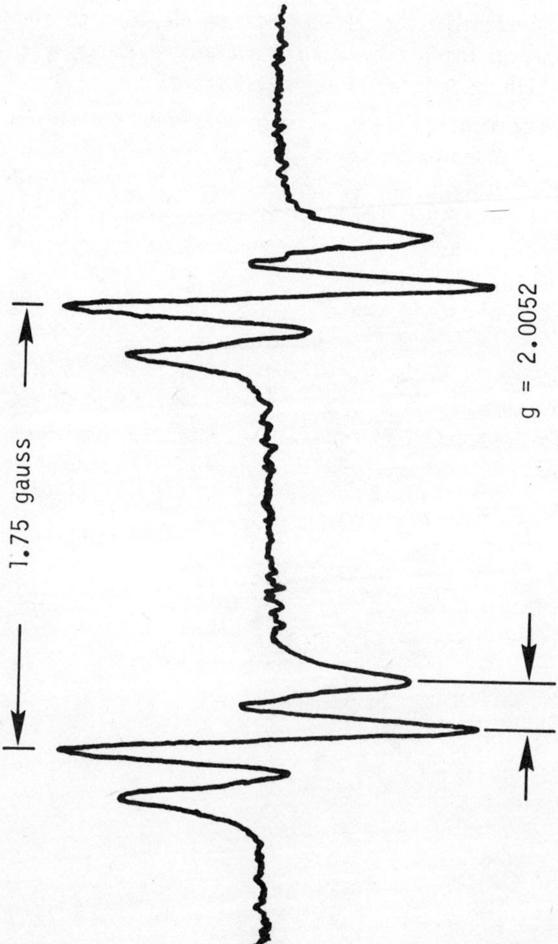

Figure 12 ESR signal of ascorbate free radical.

the two. Evidently, the MG passes an electron to the ascorbic radical formed by donating a whole electron to oxygen, which made it into a strong acceptor.

These experiments allow us to put together tentatively the chemical machinery responsible for the electronic desaturation of protein. MG added to protein attaches itself to the NH_2 groups of the lysine residues, present at the ends of the side chains. The binding between the two may be acetal-like, or may correspond to a Schiff base formed by the two. The ascorbic acid radical attaches itself to the MG, making it into a strong acceptor. The folding of the lysine side chain brings the MG into contact with the neighboring peptide bond of the protein (Fig. 8), enabling it to desaturate the valence band, taking an electron from it. The final electron acceptor of this series of reactions is the oxygen which has made a radical out of the ascorbic acid.

Casein, treated with MG in the presence of ascorbic acid and air, gives an ESR signal which has a new component not shown by casein treated with MG in the absence of ascorbic acid. In Figure 13 this signal is marked by an arrow and indicates that the ascorbic acid has entered into the protein–MG complex.

ESR gives information about reactions in which uncoupled electrons are involved; light spectroscopy gives information about reactions which involve a change in light absorption. Since uncoupled electrons are very reactive radical formation is usually accompanied by the appearance of new, and often strong light absorption. Thus, ESR and light spectroscopy are interdependent and complementary.

Mixture of MG, amines, ascorbic acid, and O_2 gives

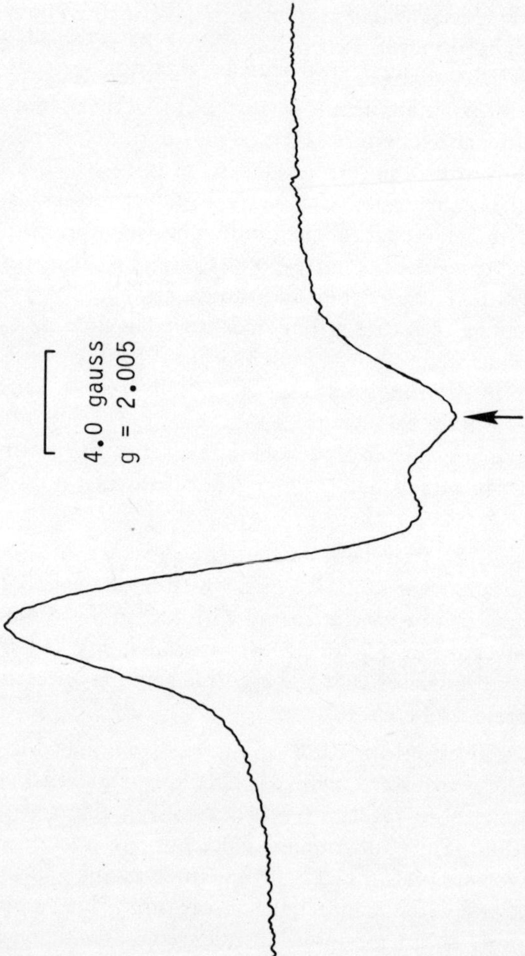

Figure 13 ESR signal of casein treated with methylglyoxal in the presence of ascorbate.

complex spectra which are very often difficult to interpret. In order to discover the role played by the individual components of a mixture one can apply differential spectroscopy. When taking the spectrum of solutions, one usually compares the absorption of the solutions in question with the absorption of the pure solvents. In differential spectroscopy one compares the absorption of a solution with the absorption of another sample of the same solution to which one more component has been added (or from which one component has been omitted). The absorption obtained is then due to the action of the one substance added or omitted.

Figure 14 shows the light absorption obtained in present research by J. McLaughlin with a solution containing 0.0033 M ascorbic acid, 0.0067 M MG, and 0.033 M methylamine. The other cuvette of the spectroscope contained the same solution without ascorbate. Both solutions had to contain O_2 since they were in open vessels. A differential spectrum was obtained which showed the absorption due to the presence of ascorbic acid. As Figure 14 shows, a high and narrow absorption peak was obtained which had its maximum at 380 nm. There was also a smaller and flatter peak with an absorption around 500 nm.

Figure 15 shows the development of the absorption over time at varied ascorbic acid concentrations. The cuvettes contained the methylamine and MG in the same concentrations as previously, but the concentration of ascorbate was varied: 0.0033 (curve 1), 0.0067 (curve 2), 0.0134 (curve 3), and 0.0267 M (curve 4). As the figure shows, the absorption increased with increasing ascorbate concentration. With the highest ascorbic acid concentration it reached maximum very quickly, and declined

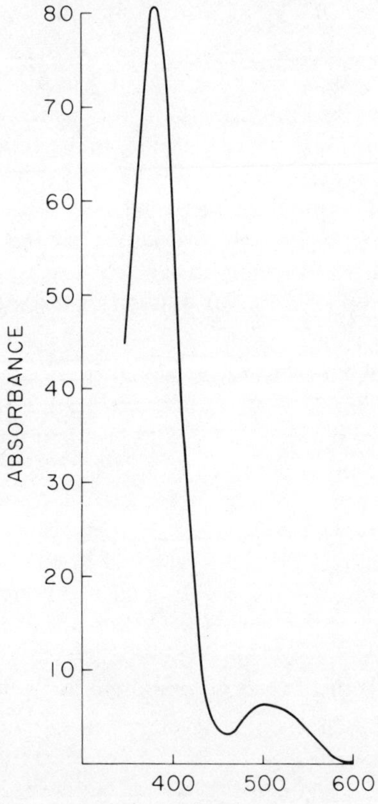

Figure 14 Absorption spectrum of a mixture of methylamine (0.033 M), methylglyoxal (0.0067 M), and ascorbic acid (0.0033 M).

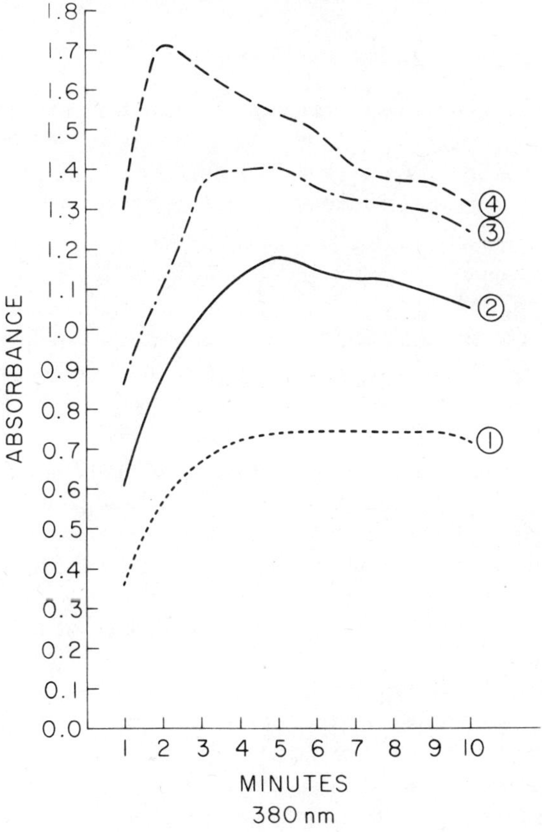

Figure 15 Absorption spectrum of a mixture of methylamine, methylglyoxal, and ascorbic acid. Concentrations of methylamine and methylglyoxal are as before; concentration of ascorbic acid, 0.0033 (curve 1), 0.0067 (curve 2), 0.0134 (curve 3), and 0.0267 (curve 4).

slowly after. The underlying reaction had to be a very rapid one.

Figure 16 shows an analogous curve in which the methylamine concentration was varied between 0.0165 (curve 1) and 0.0670 M (curve 4). Since methylamine is a base, the four curves were taken at different levels of pH.

The smaller peak in Figure 14 at 500 nm is due to the absorption of the polymer. It reaches maximum slowly (30 min) and even at its maximum is only about one-fourth as high as the peak at 380 nm. In solvents of low permittivity, such as methanol or acetone, the relation of the two peaks is reversed and the second peak at 500 nm is the high and fast one.

The absorptions shown in Figures 14 to 17 are due to the presence of ascorbate (and oxygen). If the same experiment is repeated in the absence of ascorbate and oxygen is admitted to only one of the cuvettes, a much lower and slower absorption is obtained, as shown in Figure 17. In this case both cuvettes contained a mixture of MG and methylamine and only one of the two contained oxygen. The stronger absorption and the curve were given by the cuvette which had no oxygen. The oxygen thus inhibited the reaction. The absorption obtained was due to the charge transfer obtained in the absence of oxygen. This corresponded to the situation on our globe in the α period before the appearance of oxygen. The oxygen had an inhibiting action on this charge transfer. This last experiment may be closely related to the "Pasteur effect," the inhibition of fermentation by oxygen.

As shown in Figure 15, the action of ascorbic acid increases with its increasing concentration without reach-

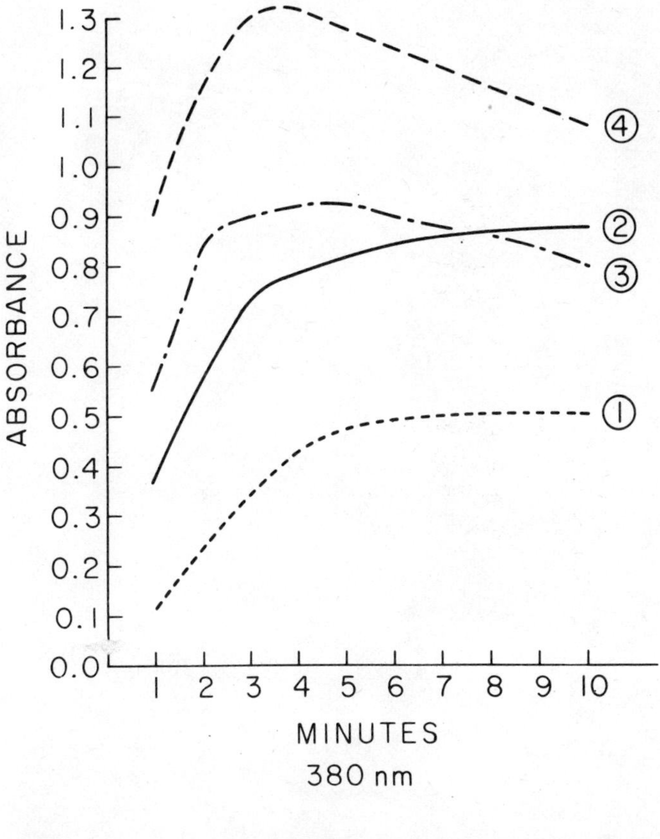

Figure 16 As Figure 14, with the concentration of methylamine varied between 0.0165 (curve 1), and 0.0670 (curve 4).

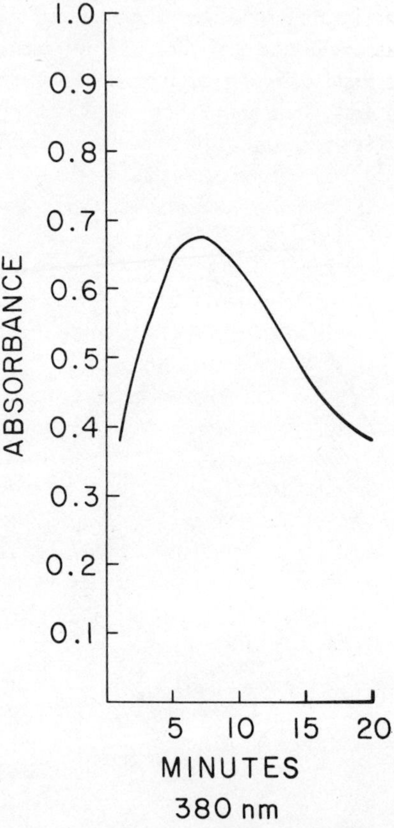

Figure 17 Absorption spectrum of a mixture of methylamine and methylglyoxal in the presence and absence of oxygen. Concentrations the same as in Figure 14.

ing a maximum within the wide limits of the experiment. This suggests an important difference between the biological action of ascorbic acid and that of other vitamins. The other vitamins have a strong biological action only when they correct a lack, an avitaminosis, and have no striking activity once the deficiency is corrected. Ascorbic acid acts stronger the more there is of it, without reaching a sharp maximum. Ascorbic acid acts at the foundation of life, transducing the protein into the desaturated living state. The more we have of it the more alive we are, a maximum being reached only with full health and vitality. The deficiency of other vitamins, which causes the failure of some specific reaction, gives rise to characteristic clinical symptoms. The lack of ascorbic acid has no characteristic symptoms short of the complete collapse known as *scurvy.* A partial lack will create only a decrease in vitality, and cause one to not eat, think, work, or love best and to not get the most fun out of life. In this state of *subscurvy* we are like a house attacked by termites: While it stands it shows no sign of weakness; its worth could be established only by exposing it to earthquakes. There are circumstances which obfuscate the situation. Since scurvy has disappeared, a lack of ascorbic acid is very rarely the direct cause of death. However, in the state of subscurvy we are more likely to get a cold, and the cold is more likely to turn into a pneumonia. If we die, our body goes to the mortuary with the diagnosis of "pneumonia" (for which we were treated). I think that many bodies go down to the mortuary with such incorrect diagnoses. A correct diagnosis of "subscurvy" would rapidly clarify the situation. When I isolated ascorbic acid I was invited to a seminar of leading German clinicians. I found them lined up against me and they sang in chorus, "There is no scurvy here and no vitamin C is needed." I had to defend myself as if I had done something wrong by isolating it.

The virtue of ascorbic acid has become its handicap. It is promoted by some of its advocates, such as I. Stone and L. Pauling, as a cure-all. This decreases confidence, since as a rule cure-alls belong to the realm of quackery. To act on a wide spectrum of physiological and pathological conditions, a substance would have to be involved in a very basic process that plays a role in all vital functions. Ascorbic acid is involved in such a process.

The shape of the ESR signal of casein treated with MG in the presence of ascorbic acid indicates that ascorbic acid is built into the protein, into its mechanism of electronic desaturation. This means that in order to build a healthy body ascorbic acid must be available all the time. When building a wall, the mortar has to be applied to every brick. It is impossible to build a strong wall without mortar and then correct by pouring mortar over it, as it is impossible to correct a vitamin deficiency by a few big doses. A correction of a deficiency is a slow job. We have to eat 60 g of protein daily to stay in nitrogen balance. Sixty grams is the daily turnover, and so the reshaping of the 15 kg of protein of an adult body has to take many months. An ample supply of vitamin is especially necessary in youth when we are building our body, beginning with intrauterine life. My own personal experience shows that at the other end of life, in senescence, the need for ascorbic acid increases rather than decreases.

The human race originated in the tropical jungle where the constant availability of food meant the constant availability of ascorbic acid. There was no need to synthesize ascorbic acid and so our body forgot how to make it. To understand the situation well we must bear in mind that not only does the monkey go through the jungle, but the jungle goes through the monkey in the form of food, drink, and air. This makes the monkey part and parcel of the jungle, and the jungle part and parcel of the monkey, so that the average ascorbic acid concentration in the monkey's body must equal the average ascorbic acid concentration of the living matter of the jungle.

Leaving the jungle we lost our ascorbic acid. Modern science and technology made it possible to live in full health outside the jungle also, offering ascorbic acid for 1.5 cents a gram. To take full advantage of this, ascorbic acid should be a household article, like sugar or flour, and be sold by the pound in the supermarket, instead of being sold in pills by the druggist.

8

SH-Glutathione and Methylglyoxal

Regulation always involves two antagonists. Traffic cannot be regulated by a green or a red light, only by a green *and* a red one, and both of these must be able to be switched on and off. Earlier I found evidence of the presence of a substance, in tissue extracts, which inhibited growth of inoculated cancer, and called the unknown substance *retine* (since it retarded growth). I also found a factor which seemed to promote cancer growth, which I called *promine*. I thought this was an example of the antagonism of regulators. I was neither the first nor the last to find such activities in tissue extracts, and spent a decade in futile attempts to isolate and identify them. Eventually, my research led me to MG, which is the inhibitor. The promotor may have been SH-glutathione. Since F. Hammett (1929) called Sulfhydryl (SH) the "hormone of cell division," the close relations of SH and proliferation, although not yet defined, are common knowledge. L. Egyud and I (1965) have shown that MG inhibits all cell division in concentrations which do not damage the cell, and I believe now that the carbonyl function is the universal brake of proliferation. The antagonism between the two substances, SH-glutathione and MG, can be demonstrated in the test tube. As M. P. Schubert (1936) showed many years ago, the two form a hemimercaptal, and so can neutralize one another to some extent, but to a particular extent only because the hemimercaptal is strongly dissociated (dissociation constant 2×10^{-3}) (Cliffe and Walley, 1961). The SH-glutathione linked to MG still gives all the classical reactions of free SH, but the antagonism is thereby not exhausted. Both substances are the central figures of antagonistic regulatory systems working together.

The red light for cell division is MG. It was not difficult to find its switch: It is the glyoxalase which transforms MG into D-lactic acid. If this is so, then glyoxalase has to have its own switch too. Professor T. Slater and I suspected that Nature switches off glyoxalase by enclosing the glyoxalase into vesicles, in analogy to lysosomes, but our friendly competition to find such vesicles remained negative. Now it is evident to me that the switch for glyoxalase is SH-glutathione. In the absence of which the glyoxalase is quite inactive. The glyoxalase being its coenzyme. What the switch for glutathione is I do not know, possibly its reversible oxidation to S–S, or else its "masking" may act as such.

SH-glutathione is present in the mouse in an average concentration of 10^{-3} M. The concentration of MG is more difficult to measure, but the mouse can tolerate an average concentration of 10^{-3} MG, SH-glutathione and MG seem to be tuned to one another around 10^{-3} M. An excess of SH-glutathione will activate the glyoxalase, which destroys the MG. An excess of MG will bind SH and inhibit all cell division, possibly also by inactivating "fixed SH," that is, SH linked to the protein.

The situation is a very complex one and I do not want to enter upon its discussion here. I only want to point out that, as I have shown in my previous booklet (1976), one can divide SH groups grossly into three classes: highly reactive, moderately reactive, and low reactivity. The fixed SH, that is, the SH linked to protein, seems to belong, to some extent, to the first group. These will hold MG the strongest, and it is likely that MG inhibits cell division by inactivating these SH-groups. The SH of glutathione belongs to the moderately active class, whereas the SH of various metabolic enzymes belongs to the inactive class, and so SH-glutathione can protect these enzymes against the inactivating action of MG. As is commonly known, the greatest part of fixed SH is "masked" and does not react with the common SH reagents as long as the protein is in the native state. These reagents become activated by the denaturation of the protein. Neither the mechanism nor the biological meaning of this masking is clear.

On the whole, SH solubilizes protein whereas MG makes it less soluble. SH also may dissociate the S–S links of protein, thus contributing to its dispersion and the loosening of the structure. This has to favor cell division, which involves a complete rearrangement of the cellular interior. It is easy to believe that cell division and the transition of the cell from the β into the α state are elicited by an outburst of SH-glutathione, as suggested by L. Rapkine (1929) 50 years ago.

Since there was no oxygen in the α period, the sulfur currently present in the form of SO_4 had to be present to a great extent as SH_2 contributing to the electron pressure. Since the α period was one of unbridled proliferation, the dominating SH became intimately involved in the mechanism of cell division, which makes the increased SH concentration demanded by cell division understandable. There can be no cell division without SH and its negative redox potential.

SH is also a general catalyst of the charge transfer reaction. Certain charge transfer reactions, such as those between ethylenediamine and MG, are entirely dependent on its presence. As cell division may be introduced by an outburst of SH, so interphase may be stabilized by a prevalence of MG over SH.

The concentration of SH can be decreased and that of MG can be increased in the animal's body only within very narrow limits without killing the animal. These limits can be exceeded by MG only when sulfhydryls are simultaneously injected (Szent-Györgyi, 1976).

9

Cancer

The research described in this booklet is dominated by the idea that we can control only what we understand. Cancer is a disturbance of a complex regulatory mechanism and to control it we have to understand this mechanism. There is no other way. In this mechanism the electronic desaturation of protein is a central feature. Cancer protein has a low degree of desaturation and paramagnetic susceptibility. The description of this regulatory mechanism may not be complete yet. Its inventory may still need completion before it will lead to the control of cancer. All the same, the data presented herein clearly indicate that this controlling mechanism is finite and has a well-defined structure, which justifies the hope that its complete knowledge will eventually lead to the control of cancer.

A cell is an integrated unit, so that changes in any of its components have to entail changes in the others. The degree of the electronic desaturation of protein decides the intensity of cohesive forces holding the cellular structures together, including the water structures surrounding the protein.

Except for the most highly differentiated cells, such as those of the brain, animal cells have two states: the state of rest and the state of proliferation. I have called these states the α and β states. The α state of proliferation is closely related to the state in which living systems existed before light and oxygen appeared. It makes all dividing cells similar to one another, and makes embryonic cells share many properties with the cancer cell. It is this undifferentiated state, with its low degree of electronic desaturation and low cohesive forces, which makes division possible. This proliferative state with its poor differentiation has higher entropy and lower free energy, which makes it the more stable state into which the cell tends to return. It is the ground state to which the cell will return when its organization is deranged. The cancer cell and the dividing normal cell differ mainly in their reversibility. The cancer cell is unable to rebuild its β state after it has completed its division and has to persist in the proliferative α state. In itself this proliferative state would not be pathological—it is only its timing and irreversibility which make it so. It is not pathological to be a baby, but it is pathological to become one and remain one at 50.

Since the cell is an integrated unit, its malignant transformation can be started up at any point in the system and by an infinite number of means. It can be started in the nucleus, its DNA, or in the protoplasm. A perturbation may induce changes which may promote further perturbations. A lack of MG, for instance, may lead to a situation in which production of MG is inhibited, making the process autocatalytic, and lead the cell into a vicious cycle which the cell is unable to break. Such vicious cycles may be broken from the outside as long as changes have not become constitutional. These cycles may play a major role in carcinogenesis.

The relations between the regulatory mechanism and carcinogens demand an extensive study. On the whole, any factor which inhibits charge transfer and the desaturation of protein has to be oncogenic, and any factor which promotes these must be carcinostatic. In a few instances, these relations are clear and simple, as is the case with the cancer of the bladder caused by β-naphthylamine in workers in the analine industry. The naphthylamine contained in urine binds the MG of the epithelium. Similarly, the cancer of the colon produced by feeding dimethylhydrazine in the experiments of A. E. Rogers and M. Newberne (1973) finds a simple explanation in the binding of MG. The close relationship between lung cancer and the inhaled carcinogenic hydrocarbons is equally evident, though we do not yet know the molecular mechanism by which these hydrocarbons produce cancer. Naturally, carcinogens need not necessarily act by attacking one of the members of the regulatory mechanism. A general loosening of the whole cellular structure, as may occur in senescence, may lead to the α state by deranging interrelations. Another instance of fairly clear interrelations is the cancer produced by H. Goldblatt and G. Cameron (1953) in tissue cultures by the lack of O_2, which is the final acceptor of the electrons taken from protein in its desaturation.

As I have shown in Chapter 5, charge transfer depends greatly on the dielectric properties of the medium. The medium of biological processes is water and the permittivity of water can be modified by its structuralization. In turn, the structuralization of water around proteins depends on the degree of electronic desaturation of the protein. As discussed earlier (see Table 1), electronic changes can be interfered with by high permittivity, such as that of water. In the immediate vicinity of the protein molecule, permittivity must be greatly modified by structuralization. Random water may be a strong oncogen, underlining the importance of the NMR measurements of F. W. Cope (1974), R. Damadian (1971), and C. Hazlewood (1969). As has been shown by these researchers, water of cancerous tissues differs from that of normal tissues by its low degree of structuralization.

A malignant transformation may be initiated in the nucleus or in the protoplasm. The fact that the cancerous state is inherited from parent to daughter cell is taken by many as evidence that the primary disturbance has to be in DNA. I am unable to accept this argument. An unbalanced state and a vicious circle may be transmitted from parent to daughter cell by the protoplasm also. But even if the primary seat is the nucleus, the changes in the protoplasmic organization have to be known and might be corrected by medication. In any case, as long as the problem of cancer is not fully cleared up, it would be a mistake to narrow our outlook.

How far the contents of this booklet will open new avenues of attack on cancer remains to be seen. What I would like to emphasize here is that distinction has to be made between therapy and prevention. It is an age-old experience that it is easier to prevent than to cure, and prevention is not necessarily a cure given in advance. The better the living machinery is built, the more functional are its single parts, and the better these parts are fitted together, then the better will the living machinery withstand perturbation. This means that the best cancer prevention is a careful guard of general health, full health. This has to start at an early age, if not during intrauterine life. As has been shown earlier, ascorbic acid plays an important role in the balance of health and disease.

Present medicine is lopsided. It looked at disease till it was blinded and forgot about health. In my student days I had to listen to unending lectures on all the diseases, but I cannot recall one on health. The present situation is probably no different. The ideal of present medicine is curing all disease, but "No Disease" is a negative. Full Health is positive.

Bibliography

Abdulnur, S. F. (1976) *Int. J. Quantum Chem. Quantum Biol. Symp. No. 3,* 59-64.

Bone, S., Lewis, T. J., Pethig, R., and Szent-Györgyi, A. (1978) *Proc. Natl. Acad. Sci. U.S.A. 75,* 315-318.

Bonsignore, A., Leoncini, G., Audisio, G., Zetta, G., and Ferruti, P. (1976) *Ital. J. Biol. Chem. 25,* 176-177; (1977) *26,* 163-168.

Brillouin, L. (1962) Giant molecules in semiconductors. *Horizons in Biochemistry* (M. Kasha and B. Pullman, eds.). Academic Press, New York.

Cliffe, E. E., and Walley, S. G. (1961) *Biochem J. 79,* 471-482.

Coman, D. R. (1944) *Cancer Res. 4* 625-629; (1953) *13,* 397-404; (1960) *20,* 1201-1204.

Cope, F. W. (1974) *J. Biol. Phys. 3,* 1-41.

Dakin, H. D., and Dudley, H. W. (1913) *J. Biol. Chem. 14,* 155-157.

Damadian, R. (1971) *Science,* 1151-1153.

Egyud, L., and Szent-Györgyi, A. (1965) *Proc. Natl. Acad. Sci. U.S.A. 55,* 388-393.

Fodor, G., Mujundar, R., and Szent-Györgyi, A. (1978). *Proc. Natl. Acad. Sci. U.S.A. 75,* in press.

Goldblatt, H., and Cameron, G. (1953) *J. Exp. Med. 97,* 525-552.

Hammett, F. (1929) *Protoplasma* 7, 297-322.

Hazlewood, C. F. (1969) *Nature 222,* 747-750.

Hazlewood, C. F., Chang, D. C., Medine, D., Cleveland, G., and Nichols, B. L. (1972) *Proc. Natl. Acad. Sci. U.S.A. 69,* 1478-1480.

Hopkins, F. G., and Morgan, E. J. (1948) *Biochem. J. 42,* 23-27.

Huggins, C. E. (1963) *Transfusions 3,* 483-493.

Kirano, Y., and Kwan, T. (1972) *Chem. Pharm. Bull. 20,* 2651-2660.

Lakid, J. (1978) *Proc. Natl. Acad. Sci. U.S.A. 75,* in press.

Lagerkrantz, C. (1964) *Acta Chem. Scand. 18,* 562.

Laki, K., and Ladik, J. (1976) *Int. J. Quantum Chem. Quantum Biol. Symp. No. 3,* 51-57.

Lohmann, K. (1932) *Biochem. Z. 254,* 332-354.

Neuberg, C. (1913) *Biochem. Z. 49,* 202-206.

Pauling, L. (1970) *Vitamin C and the Common Cold.* W. H. Freeman, San Francisco, California.

Pethig, R., and Szent-Györgyi, A. (1977) *Proc. Natl. Acad. Sci. U.S.A. 74,* 226-228.

Pohl, H. A., Gascoyne, P. R. C., and Szent-Györgyi, A. (1977) *Proc. Natl. Acad. Sci. U.S.A. 74,* 1558-1560.

Racker, E. (1951) *J. Biol. Chem. 196,* 685-696.

Racker, E. (1952) *Biochem. Biophys. Acta 9,* 577-578.

Rapkine, L. (1929) *C. R. Acad. Sci. 188,* 650-652; *191,* 871-874.

Riddle, V., and Lorenz, F. W. (1968) *J. Biol. Chem. 293,* 2718-2724.

Rogers, A. E., and Newberne, M. (1973) *Nature 246,* 491-492.

Schubert, M. P. (1936) *J. Biol. Chem. 114,* 341-350.

Shockley, W. (1950) *Electrons and Holes in Semiconductors.* D van Nostrand, Princeton, New Jersey.

Stone, I. (1972) *The Healing Factor: Vitamin C Against Disease.* Grosset, New York.

Szent-Györgyi, A. (1949) *Biol. Bull. 96*, 140-160.

Szent-Györgyi, A. (1976) *Electronic Biology and Cancer.* Marcel Dekker, New York.

Szent-Györgyi, A. (1977) *Proc. Natl. Acad. Sci. U.S.A. 74*, 2844-2847.

Takahashi, K. (1977) *J. Biochem. (Tokyo)*, 395-402, 401-414.

Yamazaki, I., Mason, H. S., and Piette, L. (1960) *J. Biol. Chem. 235*, 2444-2449.

Yamazoye, S. (1936) *J. Biol. Chem. (Tokyo) 23*, 319-334.

Index

About the Author

Albert Szent-Györgyi was born in Budapest in 1893, the fourth generation of a distinguished scientific family. He entered the University of Budapest in 1911 and that same year began working in research, performing anatomical studies in his uncle's laboratory. He received his M.D. from the University of Budapest in 1917 and his Ph.D. in chemistry from Cambridge University in 1927.

Dr. Szent-Györgyi made his first advances in the field of biochemistry with his work on metabolism, which he showed was based on both hydrogen and oxygen activation. He discovered the C_4 dicarbocylic acid catalysis, which forms the basis of the Krebs cycle. In 1937 he isolated and identified ascorbic acid, and for this work and for his metabolic studies he received a Nobel Prize in 1937. During the years of World War II, despite the turmoil of the times, Dr. Szent-Györgyi's studies on muscle resulted in the discoveries of actin, actomyosin, and their relations to ATP.

Since 1947, he has done his research in Woods Hole, Massachusetts, where he is Scientific Director of the National Foundation for Cancer Research. For the past twenty years, his interest has focused on cellular regulation and cancer. Convinced that cancer cannot be understood by any single approach, he organized what he calls a "laboratory without walls," which involves a group of leading research laboratories working on different lines but in the same direction and pooling their knowledge.

About the Author

In 1954 Dr. Szent-Györgyi won the Albert Lasker Award of the American Heart Association for his theory of muscle contraction. Dr. Szent-Györgyi is the author of several books, both scientific and philosophical, and a large number of papers. He is a member of the National Academy, honorary doctor of many leading universities, and a member of numerous scientific societies.